Frankincense Essential Oil

Benefits, Properties, Applications, Studies & Recipes

by Ann Sullivan

Published in USA by:

Ann Sullivan
217 N. Seacrest Blvd #9
Boynton Beach
FL 33425

© Copyright 2015

ISBN-13: 978-1545130070
ISBN-10: 1545130078

TABLE OF CONTENTS

Introduction

What are essential oils, and how might they be used for therapeutic purposes?

First things first, essential oils are natural and organic. They are derived from the significant compounds found in the plants that possess them. Seeds, bark, flower petals, stems and roots, as well as other functional parts of the plant, can all be used to extract essential oils from a given plant. All of us have experienced the aromatic properties of the plants that provide essential oils, even if we are completely unaware of what was taking place when it happened. Remember the last time you bought, or received, a dozen roses? That beautiful aroma exploding from the roses, is just a part of the aromatic properties and qualities of the essential oils that can be extracted from that particular flower. In conjunction with providing specific smells to certain plant species, essential oils also offer plants a layer of protection against diseases and possible predators. They also have a significant role to perform in the pollination procedures of the associated plant species.

Essential oils are not water based. They are actually phytochemicals consisting of the powerful fragrant compounds of the plant. Phytochemicals are the compounds that occur naturally within the plant itself. This means that there are no synthetic additives, which are common in conventional medicines. Essential oils are fat soluble; however, they do not possess the same fatty acids or lipids associated with animal or vegetable oil products. Essential oils are extremely clean, pure products that absorb into the skin almost immediately upon being touched. Essential oils are translucent when unadulterated and have a color range that spans from crystal clear to a deep and vibrant blue hue.

Here is an experiment you can try at home. Take a fresh lemon and slice it in half. Peel the rind from the fruit and squeeze it between your hands. That aromatic fruity smelling residue left behind is chock full of ingredients used to make essential oils.

Essential oils should not be confused with fragrance producing oils or perfumes. Essential oils are natural and organic and are taken directly from the plant. Perfumes and fragrance oils are either artificially created, or manufactured with synthetic solutions and do not possess the same therapeutic properties as essential oils. Essential oils are super concentrated substances, which means that a very little, usually a drop or two, will go a long way. The aromas and chemical compounds associated with essential oils allow them to provide therapeutic benefits for both physical and psychological procedures.

Essential oils are offered by a number of manufacturers and distributors around the world. They vary in price and quality, which is determined by a number of different factors. The country of origin for the plant species being used, how rare the botanical is, how much oil can be produced by a specific plant, growing climate present for the plants, and standards applied by the distiller/manufacturer, will all play a very important role in determining price and effectiveness of the essential oils being produced.

Essential oils are generally sold in small bottles or vials separately, or in slightly larger containers consisting of essential oil blends. The benefit of buying blends is that you can eliminate the need to purchase all essential oils separately. The disadvantage of buying blends is that you have no control of the mixture.

Chapter 4 will further detail past scientific research on frankincense essential oil. Now, let's get down to it – Essential Oil 101: the Basics of Frankincense.

Essential Oil Education

Origin: Frankincense, or Boswellia carterii, is an ancient and holy oil, used for thousands of years in Egypt and the Middle East. Its perhaps most famous purported recipient was Jesus, who was gifted with the oil by one of the three Wise Men who visited upon his birth. Traditional uses for frankincense include treatment of stomach issues and skin. It was also used to create kohl (black eyeliner in ancient Egypt), as well as for aromatic purposes. The sesquiterpenes that compose this oil stimulate emotion, while promoting hormone production in the pineal, hypothalamus and pituitary glands. The immune system also receives a boost from frankincense, as the oil stimulates leukocyte activity.

Description: Frankincense oil is commonly extracted through steam distillation. The resin is most often used. The oil is light yellow in color, thin in consistency, and has a somewhat mild fresh, spicy woody scent.

Uses: Beyond those applications previously mentioned, additional uses for frankincense essential oil include supporting the body's recovery and immunity from bronchitis, asthma, coughing, infection, colds, pneumonia, respiratory issues, strep, inflammation, nerve issues, ulcers, scars, stretch marks, immune stimulant, muscle tension, supports the nervous system, vertigo and cancer. When it comes to mood and emotion, frankincense can help relieve stress, anxiety, and depression. It centers and empowers the mind.

Properties: Anti-depressant, anti-catarrhal, anti-tumoral, anti-infectious, antiseptic, immune-stimulant, sedative, muscle relaxant and expectorant.

Application: Dilute 1:1 with a carrier oil(such as fractionated coconut oil). You can apply topically, inhale directly, diffuse or use as a dietary supplement.

Safety Precautions: Frankincense is generally regarded as safe by the FDA for internal consumption and so can be used as a dietary supplement. However, if pregnant, consult a physician before use. Remember to only use oils that are verified 100% pure, free from contaminants by 3rd party labs.

Fun facts: Frankincense is also known as olibanum, which is derived from the Arabic, "al-luban." This means "that which results from milking." The English derivative, "frankincense," actually came from the Bible, where it was documented as Francium incenseum, which means "real, pure or true incense." The oil is referred to in the Bible more than 50 times.

Frankincense has been valued for over five thousand years, with regular trade on the Arabian Peninsula and in North Africa.

Chapter 1:
Benefits of Frankincense Essential Oil

Frankincense oil offers a number of therapeutic benefits; but you may be wondering what these benefits are. In this chapter, we'll take a closer look at the history of frankincense and its many uses.

Cultivation of Frankincense

Frankincense is known in many circles as olibanum or "that which results from milking," which refers to the Boswellia sap's milky appearance. The four primary species of Boswellia trees from which frankincense is extracted provide various grades of frankincense resin, the qualities of which are determined by a number of factors, including the environment, climate, soil, and the time of harvesting.

Boswellia trees must be 8-10 years old in order to start extracting resin from them, as this is when they first begin resin production. To extract the resin, the bark is slashed in a process called striping. This enables the resin to bleed out of the bark, which then hardens on the trees in what are called "tears." The trees are tapped 2-3 times annually, with the highest quality and most opaque tears being produced in the last round. The diterpene, sesquiterpene, and terpene generally are higher quality in this batch. Somalia produces some of the finest frankincense resin and is one of the largest sources of frankincense for the Roman Catholic Church.

Each species or type of Boswellia tree produces its own type of resin. Some species are hardier than others. The Boswellia sacra species, for instance, can even grow out of rock, with the trunk of the tree attaching to the rock with a bulbous rooting.

The exploitation of Boswellia trees has affected a decline in global frankincense yield. This is largely due to the fact that those trees which have been tapped in excess only generate seeds which germinate at around 16%, as opposed to the non-tapped trees which germinate at over 80%. The pesky longhorn beetle has also impacted the Boswellia population, as has the reconstruction of agricultural land from the woodlands in which Boswellia thrive.

However, frankincense is far from extinction. Presently, the global production of frankincense clocks in around 1,000 tons, with its primary harvesting center residing in Somalia. Three harvesting zones exist there; the first is the Cal Madow mountain range in the west, the second is the Cal Miskeed section in the middle, and the last is the Cal Bari section in the east.

A History of Frankincense

The resin of frankincense is extracted from Boswellia trees and is so aromatic that it's traditionally been used in perfumes and incense. In fact, the name "frankincense" is derived from the Old French phrase for "high quality incense," or "franc encens."

Though the social value of aroma has declined over the centuries, frankincense was once a hot commodity primarily due to the scent alone. So valuable was its scent that it was gifted to baby Jesus by the wise men, along with myrrh and gold.

But frankincense goes much further back than Jesus; in fact, it goes back over 5000 years, to the trade days along North Africa's Arabian Peninsula. The Hebrews valued frankincense in association with the divine, and often used it in prayer and temple services in Jerusalem. Ancient Greece and Ancient Egypt sought frankincense as well. Egyptian Queen Hatshepsut (died 1458 BC) traded for frankincense, as depicted in the mural displayed on her temple. Famed Greek historian, Herodotus, knew the origin of frankincense was in south Arabia, but seemed to believe that the resin was difficult to harvest, as he recorded that it was guarded by deadly snakes. Herodotus claimed that the Arabs smoked the snakes out by burning the gum of the styrax tree. Even the Chinese received a decent amount of imported frankincense. According to Zhao Rugua, a Chinese writer, frankincense was transported by elephants to the Dashi, where it was then loaded onto ships to travel the remainder of the journey to China.

In the early 1990s, the lost city of Ubar, along "Incense Road," was rediscovered and is believed to be the primary trade route for frankincense.

Chemical Components

In order to generate the essential oil from the Boswellia tree resin, the resin must be steam distilled. This results in the oil's key chemical components, which are primarily ketones, sesquiterpenes, monoterpenes, sesquiterpenols and monoterpenoles. Additionally, frankincense essential oil is composed of about 56% acid resin, around 30-36% gum, and also contains phellandrene, and incensole acetate.

Main Properties of Frankincense Essential Oil

Along with the properties previously mentioned in the introduction, frankincense oil possesses anti-depressant, anti-catarrhal, anti-tumoral, anti-infectious, antiseptic, immune-stimulant, sedative, muscle relaxant, oral hygienic, carminative, cicatrisant, anti-aging, tonic, diuretic, anti-anxiety, uterine, vulnerary, and expectorant properties. With such a versatile range, frankincense is well equipped to fight off any pathogen in the body's path.

Frankincense, as mentioned, is composed of ketones, sesquiterpenes, monoterpenes, sesquiterpenoles and monoterpenoles. These components are what instill the enormously beneficial properties within frankincense essential oil. We'll outline these properties below.

Carminative

By preventing excess gas build up and/or removing it from the intestines, frankincense essential oil provides relief from abdominal pain, excess sweating, and uncomfortable indigestion.

Cicatrisant

Applied topically, frankincense is effective when it comes to skin treatments. The oil fades scars and other skin issues, such as acne, boils, stretch marks, and pox. It's also an incredible anti-agent, reducing the appearance of wrinkles and sun spots, tightening skin and providing an even tone. It does this by replacing old skin cells with new ones

Diuretic

If you're looking to lose water weight and reduce blood pressure, frankincense essential oil is your agent. The oil stimulates urination, promoting not only the loss of water weight, but the loss of fats, uric acid, sodium, and other body toxins.

Sedative

The anti-anxiety and sedative properties of frankincense essential oil produce a relaxing sense of calm, satisfaction, and insightful introspection. Because frankincense reduces blood pressure and stimulates the breathing passages, the ultimate outcome of these sedative properties is that the patient is calmed mentally.

Uterine

Frankincense essential oil helps regulate the menstrual cycle, as well as gynecological conditions. Furthermore, frankincense can prevent uterine cancer by regulating estrogen production, thereby decreasing the risk of uterine cyst and tumor formation after menopause.

Vulnerary

Whether you want to address an ulcer, a cut, or any internal or external wound, frankincense essential oil can be diluted with a skin cream and applied to expedite the process of healing while also protecting the wound from becoming infected.

Antioxidant

Anything high in antioxidants – whether fruit, beans, or essential oils – is a powerful advocate for your body. Antioxidants both protect against free radicals and repair their damage. What are free radicals? Free radicals are destructive chemicals that invade your body, produced by substances both inside and out. Some free radicals (or oxidants) form through normal bodily reactions, like inflammation, metabolism and aerobic respiration. Other free radicals form outside the body, but enter it due to exposure. These include harmful pollutants, toxins, smoking, drinking alcohol, X-rays, and UV rays, to name a few. Although our bodies produce their own antioxidants, these often become damaged as we grow older; thus, introducing antioxidants into our bodies allows these nutrients and enzymes to assist in chemical reactions which destroy the oxidants or free radicals. Frankincense essential oil is a moderate antioxidant, aiming to detox the body of free radicals that lead to disease.

Antiseptic

The antiseptic and disinfectant properties of frankincense essential oil can be reaped topically, applied directly to wounds, or even through burning; the smoke from the oil may help destroy airborne germs. Internal use will help prevent wounds from becoming infections, while external use will help prevent tetanus.

Astringent

For those who do not know what an astringent is, it's a chemical compound that shrinks body tissues, which means it can aid skin issues and irritations, everything from acne to insect bites. The astringent property of frankincense essential oil benefits everything from skin to hair to gums to muscles to intestines. As an astringent, frankincense is an anti-agent, combating muscle loss through the ability to strengthen. This astringent and coagulant properties also mean that diarrhea can be relieved through use of frankincense essential oil, as well as wound and cut bleeding.

Antidepressant

When it comes to psychological issues, the uplifting scent of frankincense combats negative thoughts and, thereby, depression.

Antifungal

While bacteria and viruses are plenty evil, fungi commonly lead to the most deadly infections, whether external or internal. Your ears, throat and nose are the most likely to become infected by fungi, the infections of which can be both excruciating and unsightly. If left untreated, fungal infections can kill, as they may spread to the brain. Frankincense essential oil protects against these infections and more and is particularly effective against skin infections.

Anti-inflammatory

External or internal inflammation can be reduced through the use of frankincense essential oil. For instance, if you or your patient has swollen fingers from arthritis or a swollen knee from a sport's injury, oral application of frankincense essential oil may decrease irritation or redness, while also soothing the pain that accompanies inflammation.

Emmenagogue

No need to look this one up. An emmenagogue is a menstrual stimulant for those with irregular menses. Frankincense regulates hormones, which means that this emmenagogue can also delay and/or reduce the symptoms of menopause, which include hormonal and mood imbalance, nausea, pain, headache, and fatigue.

Expectorant

Throat or respiratory infections can be prevented and relieved through the use of frankincense essential oil. Acting as an expectorant, frankincense breaks up and helps destroy the phlegm and mucus build ups that accompany sinuses or respiratory infections. Inflamed throat and lungs – and, thus, coughing – can also be relieved by the use of this oil.

Digestive

By boosting the production of absorptive enzymes, the digestibility of nutrients, and the secretion of digestive juices, frankincense essential oil aids the digestive tract significantly, which can make a great impact on your overall wellness by increasing those nutrients you absorb from food.

Common Therapeutic Uses

Used in traditional medicine from Asia to Africa, frankincense essential oil is safe for consumption or topical application and is most often used to support healthy skin and digestion. In India, frankincense is better known as "dhoop" and has often been applied in Ayurvedic therapy to treat wounds, arthritis, feminine wellness issues, and air purification. Daily burning of frankincense in the home has often been linked to wellness in Indian culture, as well as in Somali, Arabic, and Ethiopic cultures.

Oral Hygiene

Studies show that many oral wellness issues, such as mouth sores, bad breath, cavities, and toothaches, can be prevented and treated with frankincense essential oil. Rinsing your mouth with a frankincense mouthwash or brushing with frankincense toothpaste will provide your oral hygiene that therapeutic boost it needs.

Respiratory Issues

Frankincense calms coughing by ridding the lungs and respiratory tracts of phlegm. Bronchitis, congestion, asthma, and other respiratory issues can be treated with frankincense essential oil, as the oil's anti-inflammatory properties combine with the antidepressant properties to soothe the respiratory tract. The antiseptic and immune boosting properties also treat those ailments associated with respiratory infections, such as headaches, body aches, and fever.

Tonic

Frankincense essential oil benefits each of the body's systems, whether nervous, digestive, respiratory or excretory, making it an unbeatable general tonic. The oil also supports the immune system by helping the body absorb nutrients.

Skin Issues

Frankincense essential oil has long been used to address acne and other skin conditions. The antimicrobial properties of the oil are especially effective when treating aging skin, as the oil is a cicatrisant, which means it tightens the skin and evens out its tone. Use frankincense to treat acne, boils, stretch marks, pox, wrinkles and sun spots.

Combating the Common Cold

For those of us who are susceptible to seasonal cold and flu viruses (so...everyone), providing your immune system with a reliable mechanism of defense can mean the difference between illness and wellness. Frankincense essential oil protects your immune system and provides strong support when you need it most by combating fungal growth, which is what often causes the common cold.

Safety Precautions & Common Applications

Safety

Some adverse effects may evolve when using pure essential oils. Some essential oils should not be used when pregnant, for example, as they may cause miscarriage. Allergic reactions, too, may occur, especially when applied topically. Always administer an allergy test before committing fully to topical treatment. When used with other medications, essential oils may react negatively. If you are on any current prescription medications or have a chronic illness, such as high blood pressure, epilepsy or liver disease, then researching the effects of essential oils against your own personal medical history will eliminate any potentially problematic issues.

Note: Frankincense is generally regarded as safe by the FDA for internal consumption and so can be used as a dietary supplement. Dilute 1:1 with a carrier oil. You can apply topically, inhale directly, diffuse or use as a dietary supplement.

Blends

Oftentimes, essential oils are manufactured as blends of several pure oils. For instance, a recipe for a protective essential oil blend is a mix of cinnamon, clove, rosemary, and eucalyptus. This blend can be used to boost the immune system to help treat colds, viruses and flus. The downside to blends is that the more oils added to the mix, the higher the probability your patient may react negatively to the blend if he/she is prone to allergies. There is also the possibility of phototoxicity when working with blends.

Regardless of these possible effects, essential oils are a viable option for supporting the body's functions and addressing a number of conditions. Those looking to treat or maintain their own personal wellness, or that of their families, should consult with a doctor and become educated on the uses of essential oils, their natural remedies and the methods of treatment. Only then can you begin building your kit of essential oils for everyday use or for survival.

Chapter 2:
Recipes for Frankincense Essential Oil

In this chapter, we'll offer various recipes for frankincense essential oil, both for pure frankincense applications and blends. For pure treatments, we've provided the recommended application and dosage to help in addressing specific ailments, from Alzheimer's Disease bacteria to skin issues. When it comes to blends, herbalists and aromatherapists often combine frankincense essential oil with lemon, lime, orange, bergamot, myrrh, sandalwood, pine, lavender and benzoin. We'll offer some fantastic blending options in the second half of this chapter.

Pure Treatments

Alzheimer's Disease

To reduce the effects of Alzheimer's Disease, you might diffuse or dilute in a 1:1 ratio with a carrier oil and apply topically with a full-body or a foot massage. You can also add a couple drops to your patient's pillow or shirt collar.

Aneurysm

Help prevent aneurysm by steaming two drops of frankincense essential oil in a pan of water. Then remove the steaming pan from the stove, pour into a bowl, place a towel over your head and inhale. If you don't feel it's done its job the first time, you can reheat that same water and use it once more without adding more oil. You can also simply inhale directly or massage the oil into the soles of your feet.

Anxiety

Anxiety can be calmed through directly inhaling frankincense essential oil. Pour a drop into your hands, rub your palms together, cup them over your nose, and breathe. You can also add a drop of lavender essential oil for an all-calming blend.

Arthritis

To combat the pain and inflammation of arthritis,

dilute frankincense essential oil in a 1:1 ratio with a carrier oil and apply topically, massaging the oil into the joints. You can also simply diffuse or steam two drops of frankincense essential oil in a pan of water. Then remove the steaming pan from the stove, pour into a bowl, place a towel over your head and inhale. If you don't feel it's done its job the first time, you can reheat that same water and use it once more without adding more oil.

Asthma

Asthma can be addressed by steaming two drops of frankincense essential oil in a pan of water. Then remove the steaming pan from the stove, pour into a bowl, place a towel over your head and inhale. If you don't feel it's done its job the first time, you can reheat that same water and use it once more without adding more oil. You can also diffuse, inhale directly, or dilute in a 1:1 ratio with a carrier oil and apply topically, massaging into the throat and chest, as well as into the feet of your patient, especially over the arches and balls.
http://www.nlm.nih.gov/medlineplus/asthma.html

Bee Stings

To relieve bee sting pain, dilute in a 1:1 ratio with a carrier oil and apply topically over the sting. (Lavender can also be used to calm bee stings.)

Breathing

Enhance your breathing by directly inhaling frankincense essential oil. Pour a drop into your hands, rub your palms together, cup them over your nose, and breathe. You can also put a drop on a shirt collar, diffuse, or dilute in a 1:1 ratio with a carrier oil and apply topically, massaging into the chest.

Clear Skin

Promote clear skin by diluting 1-2 drops of frankincense essential oil in coconut oil and applying the moisturizer to a clean face. You can also diminish the appearance of blemishes by applying a drop to the affected area.

Concussion

Calm a concussion by steaming two drops of frankincense essential oil in a pan of water. Then remove the steaming pan from the stove, pour into a bowl, place a towel over your head and inhale. If you don't feel it's done its job the first time, you can reheat that same water and use it once more without adding more oil. You can also dilute frankincense essential oil in a 1:1 ratio with a carrier oil and apply topically, massaging into the toes and feet.

Confusion

To dispel confusion, you might diffuse or dilute in a

1:1 ratio with a carrier oil and apply behind the ears. You can also add a couple drops to your patient's pillow or shirt collar.

Coughs

Address a cough by steaming two drops of frankincense essential oil in a pan of water. Then remove the steaming pan from the stove, pour into a bowl, place a towel over your head and inhale. If you don't feel it's done its job the first time, you can reheat that same water and use it once more without adding more oil. You can also dilute frankincense in a 1:1 ratio with a carrier oil and apply topically, massaging into the chest and the soles of the feet.

Cuts & Sores

To accelerate skin repair and soothe pain, dilute frankincense essential oil in a 1:1 ratio with a carrier oil and apply topically to affected area.

Depression

Combat depression by steaming two drops of frankincense essential oil in a pan of water. Then remove the steaming pan from the stove, pour into a bowl, place a towel over your head and inhale. If you don't feel it's done its job the first time, you can reheat that same water and use it once more without adding more oil. You can also dilute frankincense in a 1:1 ratio with a carrier oil and apply topically, massaging into the soles of the feet.

Fibroids

Fibroids: Dilute frankincense in a 1:1 ratio with a carrier oil and applying topically, massaging into the reflex points of the feet. You can also place several drops into your bathwater or apply a single drop to a hot compress. http://www.nlm.nih.gov/medlineplus/uterinefibroids.html

Genital Warts

Genital Warts: Dilute frankincense in a 1:1 ratio with a carrier oil and apply topically to affected area on a daily basis.

Hepatitis

Hepatitis: Steam two drops of frankincense essential oil in a pan of water. Then remove the steaming pan from the stove, pour into a bowl, place a towel over your head and inhale. If you don't feel it's done its job the first time, you can reheat that same water and use it once more without adding more oil. You can also dilute frankincense in a 1:1 ratio with a carrier oil and apply topically, massaging into the hands and the soles of the feet every day.

Immune Stimulant

Give your immune system a leg up by regularly diffusing frankincense throughout your home, especially during cold and flu season. The scent also uplifts and boosts energy. Alternatively, you can add a couple drops to your bathwater or dilute with a carrier oil and apply topically. If you'd prefer the steam method, steam two drops of frankincense essential oil in a pan of water, remove the steaming pan from the stove, pour into a bowl, place a towel over your head and inhale. If you don't feel it's done its job the first time, you can reheat that same water and use it once more without adding more oil.

Infected Wounds

Infected Wounds: Steam two drops of frankincense essential oil in a pan of water. Then remove the steaming pan from the stove, pour into a bowl, place a towel over your head and inhale. If you don't feel it's done its job the first time, you can reheat that same water and use it once more without adding more oil. You can also diffuse or apply a single drop to warm water and soak the infected wound. http://www.nlm.nih.gov/medlineplus/bacterialinfections.html

Inflammation

Inflammation: Steam two drops of frankincense essential oil in a pan of water. Then remove the steaming pan from the stove, pour into a bowl, place a towel over your head and inhale. If you don't feel it's done its job the first time, you can reheat that same water and use it once more without adding more oil. You can also dilute frankincense in a 1:1 ratio with a carrier oil and apply topically, massaging into the affected area toward the heart.

Joint & Back Pain

Joint and Back Pain: Diluting frankincense in a 1:1 ratio with a carrier oil and applying topically, massaging into the affected area.

Liver Cirrhosis

Combat liver cirrhosis by diluting frankincense in a 1:1 ratio with a carrier oil and applying topically, massaging over both the liver and the outside of the right foot (the reflex point). You can also diffuse or inhale directly. http://www.nlm.nih.gov/medlineplus/cirrhosis.html

Lou Gehrig's Disease

Lou Gehrig's Disease can be addressed by steaming two drops of frankincense essential oil in a pan of water. Then remove the steaming pan from the stove, pour into a bowl, place a towel over your head and inhale. If you don't feel it's done its job the first time, you can reheat that same water and use it once more without adding more oil. You can also dilute frankincense in a 1:1 ratio with a carrier oil and apply topically in a full-body massage, stroking toward the heart, or over the soles of the feet. http://www.nlm.nih.gov/medlineplus/amyotrophiclaterals clerosis.html

Memory

Stimulate the memory by steaming two drops of

frankincense essential oil in a pan of water. Then remove the steaming pan from the stove, pour into a bowl, place a towel over your head and inhale. If you don't feel it's done its job the first time, you can reheat that same water and use it once more without adding more oil. You can also diffuse the oil wherever you study or work. Additionally, try inhaling directly, adding a few drops to bathwater, or diluting in a 1:1 ratio with a carrier oil and massaging into the base of the toes.

Mental Balance

Create mental balance by diffusing frankincense essential oil throughout your home. You can also inhale directly or dilute in a 1:1 ratio with a carrier oil and massage into the feet.

Mental Fatigue

To combat mental fatigue, place a few drops into your bathwater, or dilute in a 1:1 ratio with a carrier oil and massage into your chest or scalp.

Miscarriage (Post)

Following a miscarriage, prepare a bath with a few drops of frankincense essential oil. You can also diffuse or dilute in a 1:1 ratio with a carrier oil and massage into the abdomen and over the ankles and feet.

Moles

Reduce the appearance of moles by applying frankincense essential oil directly to the mole 3-4 times every day.
http://www.nlm.nih.gov/medlineplus/moles.html

MRSA

Combat MRSA by diluting frankincense essential oil in a 1:1 ratio with a carrier oil and applying topically to the soles of the feet and over the chest. You may also diffuse or steam two drops of frankincense essential oil in a pan of water. Then remove the steaming pan from the stove, pour into a bowl, place a towel over your head and inhale. If you don't feel it's done its job the first time, you can reheat that same water and use it once more without adding more oil.
http://www.nlm.nih.gov/medlineplus/mrsa.html

Multiple Sclerosis

Soothe multiple sclerosis with a massage. Dilute frankincense essential oil in a 1:1 ratio with a carrier oil and apply topically over the entire body or the soles of the feet. You may also diffuse or steam two drops of frankincense essential oil in a pan of water. Then remove the steaming pan from the stove, pour into a bowl, place a towel over your head and inhale.

Nasal Polyp

To combat nasal polyp, steam two drops of frankincense essential oil in a pan of water. Then remove the steaming pan from the stove, pour into a bowl, place a towel over your head and inhale. You can also dilute frankincense essential oil in a 1:1 ratio with a carrier oil and apply daily over the base of toes.

Nerve Virus

Nerve Virus: Dilute frankincense essential oil in a 1:1 ratio with a carrier oil and applying topically over the entire body or the soles of the feet, always massaging toward the heart. You can also add a few drops to bathwater.

Parkinson's Disease

The effects of Parkinson's Disease can be addressed by steaming two drops of frankincense essential oil in a pan of water. Then remove the steaming pan from the stove, pour into a bowl, place a towel over your head and inhale. Do this twice a day. You may also dilute frankincense essential oil in a 1:1 ratio with a carrier oil and apply daily as a full-body massage or over the soles of the feet.

Plague

To combat the plague, inhale directly, diffuse or dilute frankincense essential oil in a 1:1 ratio with a carrier oil and apply to the reflex points on your feet every day.

http://www.nlm.nih.gov/medlineplus/plague.html

Postpartum Depression

To combat postpartum depression, dilute frankincense essential oil in a 1:1 ratio with a carrier oil and massage into feet or apply to scalp. You can also diffuse, inhale directly, or place a few drops in your bathwater.

Scarring

Prevent scarring by adding a drop of frankincense essential oil to wounds. You can also treat acne scarring by diluting the oil in a 1:1 ratio with a carrier oil and applying to your face or skin daily. This will diminish the appearance of scars.

Stress

Relieve stress by diluting frankincense essential oil in a 1:1 ratio with a carrier oil and massaging into the soles of the feet. You can also apply directly behind the ears.

Tumor (Lipoma)

Tumors: Steam two drops of frankincense essential oil in a pan of water. Then remove the steaming pan from the stove, pour into a bowl, place a towel over your head and inhale. Do this every day. Or you can dilute frankincense essential oil in a 1:1 ratio with a carrier oil and apply topically toward the heart in a full-body massage or into your feet's reflex points.

Ulcers

Ulcers: Place a drop in each meal and take internally, or diluting frankincense essential oil in a 1:1 ratio with a carrier oil and applying topically, massaging into your feet's reflex points.

Vision

Help clarify vision by diluting frankincense essential oil in a 1:1 ratio with a carrier oil and applying topically, massaging into your the reflex points of your hands and feet. (Note: DO NOT put oils directly in or apply near the eyes.)

Warts

Rid yourself of warts through direct daily topical application of frankincense essential oil to affected area.

Wrinkles

Reduce the appearance of fine lines and wrinkles by diluting frankincense essential oil in a 1:1 ratio with a carrier oil and applying to the affected area in circular motions.

Blends

Acne Paste

Ingredients

- 1 drop German Chamomile Essential Oil

- 1 drop Myrrh Essential Oil

- 1 drop Frankincense Essential Oil

- 1 Egg White

- 1 tsp Jojoba Oil

- 1 tsp Cornflour

- 1 Tbsp Kaolin Clay

- 1 Tbsp Oats

Directions

In a small bowl, beat egg white and add in all oils, mixing until well combined. Add in other ingredients, stirring until a thick paste is formed. Apply acne paste to face and neck. Allow to sit for 30 minutes. Wash off with warm water.

Acne Serum

Ingredients

- 2 drops German Chamomile Essential Oil
- 5 drops Cypress Essential Oil
- 5 drops Frankincense Essential Oil
- 7 drops Tea Tree Essential Oil
- 3 Tbsp Hazelnut Oil

Directions

Combine all ingredients in a small dark jar or container. Close lid tightly and shake well. Apply acne serum daily to face and neck, shaking blend well before each use.

Calming Mood Mist

Ingredients

- 1 drop Frankincense Essential Oil

- 2 drops Bergamot Essential Oil

- 3 drops Lavender Essential Oil

- 4 ounces Distilled Water

Directions

Combine all ingredients in a small spray bottle. Tighten the lid and shake well. Spray into the air whenever you're in need of calm and relaxation. Shake well before each use.

Calming Rub

Ingredients

- 1 drop Lavender Essential Oil
- 1 drop Frankincense Essential Oil
- 2 drops Rose Essential Oil
- 2 drops Sandalwood Essential Oil
- 2 drops Geranium Essential Oil
- 1 tsp Carrier Oil

Directions

Combine all ingredients in a small jar or bowl. When in need of calm and relaxation, massage the calming rub into the soles of the feet.

Calming Rub II

Ingredients

2 drops Ylang Ylang Essential Oil

6 drops Frankincense Essential Oil

8 drops Clary Sage Essential Oil

1 tsp Carrier Oil

Directions

Combine all ingredients in a small jar or bowl. When in need of calm and relaxation, massage the calming rub into the soles of the feet or use for a full-body massage.

Chest Congestion

Ingredients

- 1 drop Frankincense Essential Oil

- 1 drop Peppermint Essential Oil

- 2 drops Eucalyptus Essential Oil

Directions

Steam essential oils in a pan of water. To relieve chest pain, remove the steaming pan from the stove, pour into a bowl, place a towel over your head and inhale.

Cleansing Facial Compress

Ingredients

1 drop Frankincense Essential Oil

1 drop Clary Sage Essential Oil

1 drop Sandalwood Essential Oil

Directions

Wash your face with warm water. Combine all ingredients in a small jar or bowl. Add enough warm water to soak washcloth. To cleanse, apply the warm wet washcloth to your face. Press gently and let air dry.

Face Cream

Ingredients

- 3 drops Frankincense Essential Oil

- 1 drop Lemon Essential Oil

- 1 Tbsp Aloe Vera Gel

- 1 Tbsp Beeswax

- 1/8 cup Distilled Water

- 1/8 cup Lanolin

- 1/8 cup + 2 tsp Apricot Kernel Oil

- 1/8 cup + 2 tsp Jojoba Oil

Directions

In a small bowl, combine all oils with aloe vera, mixing until well blended. Set aside. Place a mason jar in a saucepan filled with one inch of water. Over low-medium heat, put the lanolin and beeswax in the jar and stir until it melts. Remove from heat Add in distilled water and aloe vera-oil combo, stirring until a thick mixture is formed. Allow mixture to cool in the jar before use. Apply face cream daily to face and neck.

Immune Booster

Ingredients

2 drops Frankincense Essential Oil

2 drops German Chamomile Essential Oil

2 drops Ginger Essential Oil

1 drop Cinnamon Essential Oil

1 tsp Carrier Oil

Directions

Combine all ingredients in a small jar or bowl. During cold and flu season, massage the immune boosting rub into the soles of the feet.

Meditative Diffusing Blend

Ingredients

- 6 drops Frankincense Essential Oil

- 5 drops Patchouli Essential Oil

- 4 drops Sandalwood Essential Oil

- 2 drops Sandalwood Essential Oil

- 2 drops Geranium Essential Oil

- 1 Tsp Carrier Oil

Directions

Combine all ingredients in a diffuser for a mind-balancing meditative blend.

Moisturizer for Normal Skin

Ingredients

- 8 drops Palmarosa Essential Oil

- 12 drops Frankincense Essential Oil

- 25 drops Lavender Essential Oil

- 3 ounces Almond Oil

- 1 ounce Jojoba Oil

Directions

Combine all ingredients in a small jar or bowl. Apply moisturizer to your face each morning and night.

Tension Headache

Ingredients

- 1 drop Lavender Essential Oil
- 1 drop Frankincense Essential Oil

Directions

Combine oils and rub into your temples and your forehead to reduce tension or headache.

Chapter 3:
Frankincense Essential Oil Studies

Many studies have been done on essential oils to discover and prove their therapeutic qualities. In the case of the great number of frankincense studies, many of the properties attributed to the essential oil (noted in this book and elsewhere) are quite often validated through the scientific research of accredited universities and published by accredited scientific journals. In this chapter, we'll discuss a small portion of these studies. It's important to note that research on essential oils is constant and evolving. Keep up with any recent research, as it may turn up even further valuable uses of these miracle oils. (Additional research can be found at http://www.pubmed.gov)

Study 1 – Anticancer Properties (Pancreatic Cancer)

In this study published by the BMC Complementary and Alternative Medicine, the antimicrobial effects of frankincense essential oil were examined, with the following results: "Regardless of the availability of therapeutic options, the overall 5-year survival for patients diagnosed with pancreatic cancer remains less than 5%. Gum resins from Boswellia species, also known as frankincense, have been used as a major ingredient in Ayurvedic and Chinese medicine to treat a variety of health-related conditions. Both frankincense chemical extracts and essential oil prepared from Boswellia species gum resins exhibit antineoplastic activity, and have been investigated as potential anti-cancer agents. The goals of this study are to identify optimal condition for preparing frankincense essential oil that possesses potent anti-tumor activity, and to evaluate the activity in both cultured human pancreatic cancer cells and a xenograft mouse cancer model...Human pancreatic cancer cells were sensitive to Fractions III and IV (containing higher molecular weight compounds) treatment with suppressed cell viability and increased cell death...In addition, Boswellia sacra essential oil Fraction IV exhibited anti-proliferative and pro-apoptotic activities against pancreatic tumors...All fractions of frankincense essential oil from Boswellia sacra are capable of suppressing viability and inducing apoptosis of a panel of human pancreatic cancer cell lines. Potency of essential oil-suppressed tumor cell viability may be associated with the greater abundance of high molecular weight compounds in Fractions III and IV. Although chemical component(s) responsible for tumor cell cytotoxicity remains undefined, crude essential oil prepared from hydrodistillation of Boswellia sacra gum resins might be a useful alternative therapeutic agent for treating patients with pancreatic adenocarcinoma, an aggressive cancer with poor prognosis."

According to the study, frankincense essential oil was effective in suppressing viability and stimulating apoptosis in human pancreatic cancer cell lines. In multicellular organisms, apoptosis is the process of programmed cell death. In the case of cancer, an insufficient amount of apoptosis results in an unmanageable growth of cancer cells, so the cell death induced by frankincense essential oil is necessary to controlling the cancer. The study shows that frankincense may be beneficial to those with pancreatic cancer.

http://www.ncbi.nlm.nih.gov/pubmed/23237355
http://www.ncbi.nlm.nih.gov/pmc/articles/PMC3538159/pdf/1472-6882-12-253.pdf

Study 2 – Anticancer Properties (Breast Cancer)

In this study published by the Oncology Letters, the anticancer effects of frankincense essential oil were examined, with the following results: "The present study aimed to investigate the composition and potential anticancer activities of essential oils obtained from two species, myrrh and frankincense...The results indicated that the MCF-7 and HS-1 cell lines showed increased sensitivity to the myrrh and frankincense essential oils compared with the remaining cell lines. In addition, the anticancer effects of myrrh were markedly increased compared with those of frankincense, however, no significant synergistic effects were identified. The flow cytometry results indicated that apoptosis may be a major contributor to the biological efficacy of MCF-7 cells."

MCF-7 is a breast cancer cell line. When the cell line is broached by frankincense or myrrh essential oils, the result is cell death. In multicellular organisms, apoptosis is the process of programmed cell death. In the case of cancer, an insufficient amount of apoptosis results in an unmanageable growth of cancer cells, so the cell death stimulated by frankincense essential oil is necessary to control the cancer.

http://www.ncbi.nlm.nih.gov/pubmed/24137478

http://www.ncbi.nlm.nih.gov/pmc/articles/PMC3796379/pdf/ol-06-04-1140.pdf

Study 3 – Anticancer Properties (Breast Cancer)

In this study published by the BMC Complementary and Alternative Medicine, the anticancer effects of frankincense essential oil were examined, with the following results: "Essential oil prepared by distillation of the gum resin traditionally used for aromatic therapy has also been shown to have tumor cell-specific anti-proliferative and pro-apoptotic activities. The objective of this study was to optimize conditions for preparing Boswellia sacra essential oil with the highest biological activity in inducing tumor cell-specific cytotoxicity and suppressing aggressive tumor phenotypes in human breast cancer cells...Western blot analysis was performed to study Boswellia sacra essential oil-regulated proteins involved in apoptosis, signaling pathways, and cell cycle regulation...All three human breast cancer cell lines were sensitive to essential oil treatment with reduced cell viability and elevated cell death, whereas the immortalized normal human breast cell line was more resistant to essential oil treatment. Boswellia sacra essential oil...inducing cancer cell death, preventing the cellular network formation (MDA-MB-231) cells on Matrigel, causing the breakdown of multicellular tumor spheroids (T47D cells), and regulating molecules involved in apoptosis, signal transduction, and cell cycle progression...Similar to our previous observations in human bladder cancer cells, Boswellia sacra essential oil induces breast cancer cell-specific cytotoxicity. Suppression of cellular network formation and disruption of spheroid development of breast cancer cells by Boswellia sacra essential oil suggest that the essential oil may be effective for advanced breast cancer. Consistently, the essential oil represses signaling pathways and cell cycle regulators that have been proposed as therapeutic targets for breast cancer."

This study, again, examined the effect of frankincense essential oil on breast cancer cells with much the same results as the first study. Beyond the previous study, the results indicate that frankincense essential oil may be effective in combatting advanced breast cancer, due to its ability to suppress the cellular network formation and disrupt spheroid development of breast cancer cells.

http://www.ncbi.nlm.nih.gov/pubmed/22171782

http://www.biomedcentral.com/1472-6882/11/129

Study 4 – Antimicrobial Properties

In this study published by the Letters to Applied Microbiology, the antimicrobial effects of frankincense essential oil were examined, with the following results: "To evaluate the anti-biofilm activity of the commercially available essential oils from two Boswellia species...the essential oil of Boswellia papyrifera showed considerable activity against both Staphylococcus epidermidis DSM 3269 and Staphylococcus aureus ATCC 29213 biofilms...Boswellia rivae essential oil was very active against preformed C. albicans ATCC 10231 biofilms and inhibited the formation of C. albicans biofilms at a sub-MIC concentration...Essential oils of Boswellia spp. could effectively inhibit the growth of biofilms of medical relevance."

Staphylococcus epidermidis and Staphylococcus aureus are both Gram-positive bacterium. Although Staphylococcus epidermidis is part of the normal human skin flora and is not typically pathogenic, those with compromised immune systems can potentially develop an infection from the bacteria. Staphylococcus aureus is also commonly found on the skin and in the respiratory tract, and is not always pathogenic. But, when it becomes so, S. aureus produces respiratory issues like sinusitis, skin infections, and even food poisoning. This study tested a species of frankincense against these biofilms and found that the essential oil actively combated both strains of bacteria.

http://www.ncbi.nlm.nih.gov/pubmed/19146534

http://www.ncbi.nlm.nih.gov/pmc/articles/PMC2664784/

Study 5 – Anti-inflammatory Properties

In this study published by the Indian Journal of Pharmaceutical Sciences, the anti-inflammatory effects of frankincense essential oil were examined, with the following results: "The resin of Boswellia species has been used as incense in religious and cultural ceremonies and in medicines since time immemorial. Boswellia serrata

(Salai/Salai guggul), is a moderate to large sized branching tree of family Burseraceae (Genus Boswellia), grows in dry mountainous regions of India, Northern Africa and Middle East...The resinous part of Boswellia serrata possesses monoterpenes, diterpenes, triterpenes, tetracyclic triterpenic acids and four major pentacyclic triterpenic acids i.e. β-boswellic acid, acetyl-β-boswellic acid, 11-keto-β-boswellic acid and acetyl-11-keto-β-boswellic acid, responsible for inhibition of pro-inflammatory enzymes. Out of these four boswellic acids, acetyl-11-keto-β-boswellic acid is the most potent inhibitor of 5-lipoxygenase, an enzyme responsible for inflammation."

This study took a look at the chemical composition of the Boswellia serrata species of frankincense essential oil. The study found that frankincense contains four boswellic acids, one of which is acetyl-11-keto-β-boswellic acid. The enzyme which produces inflammation (5-lipoxygenase) is inhibited by this particular acid, which is what makes the essential oil of frankincense effective as an anti-inflammatory.

http://www.ncbi.nlm.nih.gov/pubmed/22457547

http://www.ncbi.nlm.nih.gov/pmc/articles/PMC3309643/

Study 6 – Immune Support

In this study published by the Department of Pharmacognosy at Mansoura University in Egypt, the microbial and immune supportive effects of frankincense essential oil were examined, with the following results: "The yield of steam distillation of frankincense essential oil (3%); and its physicochemical constants were determined...Biologically, the oil exhibited a strong immunostimulant activity (90% lymphocyte transformation) when assessed by a lymphocyte proliferation assay."

The lymphocyte transformation test (LTT) is an in vitro immunity test which determines the proliferation of T cells to an antigen (in this case, frankincense) in vitro. The uptake of radioactive thymidine by the lymphocytes is what measures the transformation, as this uptake demonstrates protein synthesis. In the case of frankincense essential oil, the LTT revealed that the oil was an effective immunostimulant, with 90% lymphocyte transformation.

http://www.ncbi.nlm.nih.gov/pubmed/12710734

Chapter 4:
The Ins & Outs of Essential Oils

Where do essential oils come from?

Plants and plant species naturally produce essential oils for various reasons, one being to draw pollinator insects to them, another being to repel invading organisms (bacteria, animals). A number of chemical compounds compose each plant's essential oil, and the combination of these compounds is specific to each oil, which then instills in the oil its own unique properties. Essential oils can be harnessed from all sorts of plant components, including flowers, leaves, bark, fruit, roots, and resin. For instance, cinnamon oil is harnessed from bark, lemon oil from the peel, and lavender oil from lavender flowers. Certain plants can produce a few chemical variants of the same essential oil, which are acquired from different parts of the plant.

Some of these parts produce a large amount of oil, while others produce just a smidgen. The oil's quality and potency depends upon a number of factors, including the subspecies of the plant, its soil conditions, the time of year and even the time of day you harvest it.

How are essential oils extracted?

Essential oils can be extracted from plants through various methods, including pressing, distillation, solvent and maceration. Let's take a brief look at each:

Pressing Method

Commonly used with citrus fruit, the pressing method extracts the oil through a technique which involves pushing the fruit peels through a press. Oily fruits and plants are best suited for this technique. Orange oil, for example, is extracted from orange skins through the pressing method.

Distillation Method

This technique harkens back to the days of old-timey moonshiners, as the same sort of method used to create strong liquor can be used to extract essential oils. Using a still, boiled water and plant materials will create steam which is then cooled by coils and condensed into a combination of water and oil. This combination doesn't mix, so the oil can then be extracted from it.

Solvent Method

Through a multi-step process, certain plant and flower oils can be extracted using alcohol and other solvents, which extort the essential oil from the plant materials.

Maceration Method

When a "carrier" or fixed oil or lard is mixed with the plant material and set out in the sun, over a period of time, the carrier oil is infused with the plant's essence. Heat sources, other than the sun, are often used to speed the process. Throughout the process, more plant material is added to produce a more potent oil.

How do you use essential oils?

Although some studies about the effectiveness of essential oils are conducted by small companies or even individuals, a number of them are conducted by the food and cosmetic industries. In general, the pharmaceutical industry shows next to no interest in herbal medicine, primarily because there are few options to patent such products. Being as such, the product's lack of profitability results in a lack of research funding. Regardless, the historical uses of essential oils tell us what we need to know: these oils have been effectively administered for centuries. The therapeutic qualifications of essential oils can be plotted in the survival of the human race across cultures and generations.

Another reason that studies on essential oils have not resulted in much conclusive evidence as to their overall effectiveness is because definitive results are sometimes difficult to prove, as the quality of each batch of oil can vary for a number of reasons. One is that essential oils are impossible to standardize. As mentioned above, even the slightest variance in soil conditions and the time of harvesting – as well as innumerable other factors – will produce a different product quality and potency. In addition, essential oils are often obtained from various species of the same plant; Eucalyptus radiata and Eucalyptus globulus can both be used in the making of therapeutic-grade eucalyptus oil and, as a result, they may have slightly different properties and degrees of strength or effectiveness.

Just as there are a number of methods by which to extract essential oils, there are a number of methods to administer them therapeutically. The variety of chemical compounds in each essential oil means that their benefits and applications also vary across the board. Below are a few of these methods.

Topical Administration

Direct application of many essential oils works like a sponge, as skin sops up chemicals and other things (like sunlight, for instance). Topical application is best when you want to clear up an ailment on the skin's surface or in the underlying muscle tissue. When applying topically, you may either massage the oil into the skin or simply dab on the skin for therapeutic results. You might combine the essential oil with a carrier oil for topical use in order to dilute its potency. This is safer, as the oil is so concentrated. You may support your body's defenses against rash or muscle pain in this manner, but you should always test your patient for allergies before applying. Adverse effects are produced by natural chemicals as much as synthetic ones; poison ivy, for example.

To test for allergens, place a drop or two on your patient's inner forearm. If a rash develops within 12 to 24 hours, then the patient is allergic. In addition, phototoxicity – sun exposure resulting in an exacerbated burn – may be an issue when citrus oils are applied topically. So one must proceed with caution when applying essential oils using this method.

Inhalation Therapy

Commonly known as "aromatherapy", this essential oil application is effective for inner ailments, like sore throat or cold. In a steaming bowl of distilled or sterilized water, add a few drops of essential oil and, with a towel over your head, bend over the bowl and inhale. The towel captures the vapors, making the technique even more effective. Essential oils can also be placed in a diffuser or potpourri throughout a room to produce somewhat diluted therapeutic effects.

Ingestion

When using this method, proceed with caution. Direct ingestion of essential oils must be monitored and applied in small doses that are diluted in a tablespoon or more of any carrier oil – olive oil, for example. If you are unsure of dosage amounts, make a tea with the relevant herb instead. Although the effects of this diluted use may be weaker, this application is a better alternative than an overdose of essential oils.

What are the general benefits of using essential oils?

Replacement for Prescription Drugs

One practical benefit for using essential oils is, of course, their substitutive nature; they can replace Rx drugs, which is the ultimate reason to educate yourself on their administration and to begin stockpiling your essential oil supply. One of the potential threats of economic or social collapse is the lack of resources, and primarily the inability to procure prescription drugs. Being as such, finding suitable supplements should be a priority when preparing for the worst.

Their portability is also a major bonus when it comes to survival prepping. The fact that these ultra-concentrated oils take up little-to-no space makes toting them to your shelter all the simpler should the need arise. And, because essential oils are highly concentrated, the application used in most methods of administration requires only a drop or two of oil, which means that tiny bottle will be long-lasting.

Cost Effective Supplement

Though money may be the last thing on your mind when it comes to prepping for a survival situation (money may even be obsolete in the event of social collapse), it is worth noting that the expense of essential oils pales in comparison to prescription drugs. Essential oils are a cost effective supplement to prescription medicine.

No Expiration Date

Another benefit of essential oils is that they do not expire, neither do they have "proper storage" requirements. A number of medicines and medicinal products must be replaced every couple years, so this sets essential oils ahead of the pack when it comes to shelf life.

Versatility

Essential oils also offer great versatility. Apart from providing therapeutic benefits, essential oils can be repurposed for household and hygienic applications. For instance, if you're looking for something that might serve your dental hygiene needs in a time of crisis, the protective oil blend is your go-to essential oil. If you want to maintain your skin's tone and condition, frankincense and lavender will do the trick; the latter also serves as sunscreen, so you can inhibit sun damage as well.

When it comes to the house or shelter, you can use essential oils to deodorize, which will come in handy in a disaster scenario where things might start to smell fishy due to lack of proper utilities and care. For example, after the 2011 tsunami and the subsequent nuclear reactor meltdown in Japan, a nurse named Risa Nakahira used essential oils to deodorize and sanitize putrid public bathrooms in overpopulated evacuation facilities. As relief workers searched for survivors, often wading through debris and decay, Nakahira also deodorized their boots and masks using essential oils. The possibilities of these natural oils are endless.

They are also versatile when it comes to the range of patients they're capable of supporting. The wellness of everyone from your great grandfather to your infant baby can be fortified with the aid of essential oils in the appropriate dosage. They even come in handy when supporting the wellness of livestock or pets. From teething infants to dementia in the elderly, from teenagers with acne to dogs with urinary tract infections, essential oils can serve any patient with nearly any ailment.

Conclusion

Now that you know all about what frankincense essential oil can do for you – where it originates, how it's extracted, its benefits and properties, and the different methods of administration – you can use it confidently to treat wellness issues and start to assemble a kit of essential oils for survival or to be used in day to day life!

Essential oils can be purchased online or at your local holistic treatment store – be sure they are 100% pure and can be taken internally before you buy.

The various benefits of essential oils and their properties are countless. To build your own kit, first focus on acquiring the essential oils which may bear more relevance to your wellness issues or the potential threats within your environment or invest in a kit with multiple oils.

In the event of a viral outbreak, for instance, frankincense essential oil will be one of your more crucial oils due to their antiviral and immuno-supportive properties.

Used as a supplement or as your go-to treatment for skin conditions, viral infections or immune-boosting agents, the application of frankincense essential oil in medicine has survived for centuries and will survive centuries more. When it comes down to it, you don't need to rely solely on pharmaceuticals; essential oils, herbs, and plenty of other natural ingredients can be used to help treat any number of wellness issues, whether ailment or injury.

Essential oils are essential to your survival in the case of viral outbreak, social collapse or natural disaster because, when the SHTF, your access to pharmaceuticals will likely either be limited or eliminated altogether. Supplements to our modern-day standard will equate survival when no other option exists. And when it comes to a life-or-death situation, you can't let your wellness decline, no matter the state of the world

DISCLAIMER AND/OR LEGAL NOTICES: Every effort has been made to accurately represent this book and it's potential. Results vary with every individual, and your results may or may not be different from those depicted. No promises, guarantees or warranties, whether stated or implied, have been made that you will produce any specific result from this book. Your efforts are individual and unique, and may vary from those shown. Your success depends on your efforts, background and motivation.

The material in this publication is provided for educational and informational purposes only and is not intended as medical advice. The information contained in this book should not be used to diagnose or treat any illness, metabolic disorder, disease or health problem. Always consult your physician or healthcare provider before beginning any nutrition or exercise program. Use of the programs, advice, and information contained in this book is at the sole choice and risk of the reader.